Contents

So Easy Baby Food
Homemade Baby Food in Less Than 30 Minutes Per Week

Published by Fresh Baby LLC
202 Grove Street, Petoskey, MI 49770
www.freshbaby.com

ISBN: 9780-97-272275-9

Author: Cheryl Tallman
Cover and Book Design: Dylan Tallman, Creative i
Photography: Roger Tallman, Creative i
Editor: Jillian Lieder

Healthy Eating Habits

Introducing solid food begins when your baby is about 6 months old. Solid food is, at first, an add-on to the main source of nutrition, breast milk or infant formula. Until your baby is 12 months old, solid food remains a secondary source of nutrition. If you don't know much about healthy eating, don't worry. You have about 6 months to begin learning. There is no better way to learn what's healthy than to make baby food at home.

Teaching your child healthy eating habits will have lifetime benefits. There is no better time to start than with the first bites of solid foods. Having healthy eating habits does not mean dieting. Unless your baby's diet is being watched by a healthcare provider, you do not need to count calories or choose low-fat or non-fat foods. It is really quite simple to form healthy eating habits. Here are some tips to get you started:

1. **Be a good role model.** Babies learn through watching you and others around them. Be a positive force for your baby by eating healthy foods, such as fruits and vegetables. Remember, your baby will respond to what you like.

2. **Don't give up.** Babies' tastes change daily. The fact that your baby spits out peas one day does not mean he doesn't like them. Unless he has shown signs of an allergic reaction, try the food again in a couple days—you may be pleasantly surprised.

3. **Offer variety.** All foods contain different vitamins and nutrients. Eating many types of foods will lead to a balanced diet. When your baby first starts eating, the amount is not as important as the variety.

4. **Encourage drinking water.** Water helps the body digest foods. As your baby is introduced to solid food, the need for water is greater. At about 8 or 9 months old, offer your baby 2 to 3 ounces of water at each meal.

5. **Don't be in a rush.** Many babies are slow eaters. At the beginning feeding time may go REALLY slowly. Allow plenty of time for meals so you and your baby can relax and enjoy your time.

6. **Never force babies to eat or to finish all their food.** Your baby will eat when she is hungry. And she will eat the types of foods her body needs most. During meals allow her to eat as much or as little as she wants.

7. **Avoid distractions.** Make mealtimes a family event. The whole family should eat together any time you can. This will help your baby learn to interact with others at mealtime and to begin developing social skills.

8. **Be positive about vegetables and fruits.** Let your baby know what he is eating when you are feeding him. Talk about the vitamins he is getting and about how important they are for growing bigger and stronger.

Introducing Solid Foods

The American Academy of Pediatrics recommends the introduction of solid food at about 6 months of age. The introduction to solid food is a very important step in your baby's development. Making baby food is a great way to make sure that your baby is getting the best in quality, nutrition, and taste.

Fruits and Vegetables—One at a Time

As you start to introduce solid food, it is very important to watch out for allergic reactions to new foods. It is best to introduce foods slowly. There is really no reason to rush. You can simply follow the "One at a Time" plan: feed only one food to your baby for 3 to 5 days. This will allow enough time to see whether your baby has any allergies to the food. Once you know that your baby does not react to a food, you can move on to another one.

Food Allergies

You should discuss any food allergies in your family with your healthcare provider before giving solid food to your baby. A family history of food allergies may put your baby at higher risk. This just means that you may have to try foods in a different order.

 Once you start feeding your baby new foods one at a time, watch for any changes in him. Food allergies can happen even if they do not run in your family. A rash is not the only sign of food allergy. Some common symptoms of food allergies include:

*   Rashes, especially on the face
*   Diaper rash
*   Hives
*   Runny nose, watery eyes, or sneezing
*   Diarrhea, gas, or vomiting
*   Fussiness or irritability
*   Temperament changes
*   Puffy eyes

If you notice any of these signs, stop feeding your baby the new food. Describe the signs to your healthcare provider. If she believes that a food allergy is the cause, be sure she writes it on your baby's health chart at her office. Most allergic reactions in babies are temporary. The problem foods can usually be reintroduced when the baby is a little older.

One way that may prevent food allergies is to delay foods that are known to cause allergic reactions. You can try them when your baby is older. Here is a list of the foods that cause allergies most commonly.

Wait until after 12 months to introduce:

- Berries
- Chocolate
- Citrus fruits (oranges, lemons, limes, etc)
- Cow's milk
- Eggs
- Fish
- Soy
- Wheat

Wait until after 3 years to introduce:

- Shellfish (shrimp, crab, clams, etc)
- Nuts
- Peanuts

Steer clear of processed foods until your baby is at least 12 months old. These foods can contain additives, artificial colors, and preservatives. These ingredients can cause allergic reactions in babies.

Foods Not Good For Babies

There are many choices of tasty, healthy foods for your baby, but not all foods are baby-friendly. Here are some foods that are not good for your baby.

Sugar, high fructose corn syrup, salt and caffeine	Delay introducing as long as possible	Avoid foods that contain these items as main ingredients.
High nitrate foods	Introduce over 8 months	Beets, carrots, green beans, spinach, and collard greens. Also hot dogs, ham, bologna, sausages, salami, and many other deli meats.
Foods that can contain disease-causing bacteria	Introduce over 12 months	Honey, un-pasteurized foods (i.e. apple cider), blue cheese, brie, and raw fish.
Frequent allergens	Introduce over 12 months, possibly much later	Berries, chocolate, citrus fruits, cow's milk, egg whites, fish and shellfish, nuts, peanuts, and tomatoes. Processed foods with additives, coloring agents, and preservatives
Choking hazards	Introduce at 2-3 years	Nuts (other than finely ground); peanut butter; caramel; candy; gum; whole grapes; raw, hard fruits and veggies; chunks of meat; pieces of bacon; hot dogs; sunflower seeds; popcorn; raisins; potato chips; and hard candy.
Hot foods	Introduce after 2-3 years	All foods should be served cold, at room temperature, or slightly warm.

Mealtime Tips for Feeding

Baby food can be served cool, at room temperature, or slightly heated. Always test the temperature of food before feeding it to your baby. If you use a microwave to warm food, stir the food thoroughly before testing the temperature.

When you first start feeding your baby, plan on sitting with him and offering food for about 20 minutes at each meal. It is okay if your baby does not finish his meal. Sometimes he will eat a lot, sometimes only a little. Don't panic, this is normal. Your baby will let you know when he is done—common signs include:

- Pushing the spoon away from his mouth
- Hitting at the spoon
- Playing with his food
- Spitting food out
- Turning his head away

Choking can occur when your baby is introduced to solid foods. Protect your baby from choking hazards by:

- Always supervising him while eating
- Feeding him only when he is in a chair or sitting down
- Not allowing him to crawl or walk around while eating
- Avoiding foods that are likely to cause choking (see "Foods not good for babies").

How much is enough?

When you begin solid foods, amount is not as important as variety. Don't worry if your baby is eating only a few spoonfuls of food at first. This is normal. Over the next few months, your baby will begin to eat more solid food. When she reaches 12 to 18 months, she'll be eating a combination of milk (either breast milk or cow's milk) and solid foods. The American Academy of Pediatrics provides the guidelines below for a baby's minimum daily food intake at about 12 to 18 months.

Food	Servings
Whole Milk	16-24 ounces
Fruits & vegetables	4-8 Tablespoons
Bread & cereals	4 servings (a serving equals ¼ slice of bread or 2 Tablespoons of rice, potatoes, pasta, etc.)
Meat, poultry, fish, eggs, beans	2 servings (a serving equals one tablespoon)

Getting Started Making Baby Food

Choosing Fruits and Vegetables for Homemade Baby Food

You can use fresh, frozen, or canned fruits and vegetables to make baby food. Buying canned or frozen food is easy, but choosing fresh produce can be tricky. Here are some shopping tips for picking the freshest items at the market:

- Choose fresh-looking fruits and vegetables that are not bruised, shriveled, moldy, or slimy.
- Don't buy anything that smells bad.
- Don't buy packaged vegetables that have a lot of liquid in the bag or that look slimy. Some fruits, such as fresh-cut pineapple, will have liquid in the bag, and that's okay.
- Buy only what you need because most fruits and vegetables are not "stock-up" items. Some, such as apples and potatoes, can be stored at home, but most items should be used within a few days.
- Handle produce carefully at the store. Keep produce on top in your shopping cart (heavy items on top will bruise fruits and vegetables, and raw meat products might drip juices on them).
- Set produce gently on the checkout belt so it doesn't bruise. Some items that may seem hardy, such as cauliflower, actually are very delicate and bruise easily.
- Wash produce just before you use it, not when you put it away.

Cooking Steps for Making Baby Food

1. Prep: Wash, chop, and peel fresh fruits and vegetables if necessary. If you are using frozen foods, simply open the package. If you are using canned foods, pour them into a colander or strainer and rinse in cold water for one minute and skip to the puree step.

2. Cook: You can cook the food in the microwave or use the stovetop to steam it. Cooking times are listed on each recipe. If a fork slides easily into the food or it can be mashed with a fork, it is ready for the next step.

3. Puree: Pour the cooked food and the juices into a blender or food processor and puree. This is the most important step in making baby food. The food should be soft and smooth for your baby.

4. Freeze: Pour the pureed food into ice cube trays and cover them. Put them in the freezer for 8 to 10 hours or overnight.

5. Pop and Store: Write the type of food and the date on a freezer storage bag. Remove the baby food trays from the freezer and quickly run hot water over the back of the tray. Twist the tray to pop the baby food cubes out and into the freezer storage bag. Place the storage bag in the freezer. Frozen baby food cubes will keep fresh for 2-3 months in the freezer.

Serving Homemade Baby Food

Baby food should always be served cool, slightly warm, or at room temperature. It is easy to get ready for a meal. Simply select baby food cubes from the freezer and place them in a dish. You can use one of these methods for thawing:

- Refrigerator: Thawing food in the refrigerator is the easiest method but requires planning ahead. Simply place a covered dish containing food cubes in the refrigerator. In about 3 to 4 hours, they will thaw. You can warm the cubes on the stove, in a hot water bath on the counter, or in the microwave.

- Microwave: Thawing food in the microwave is fast. Simply place a microwave-safe dish containing food cubes in the microwave and defrost them. Some foods defrost faster than others do. Defrosting two dishes of food at once may take a little longer.

* Warning: Microwaves create hot spots in food. When using a microwave to thaw or warm baby food, stir the food well before serving. Always check the temperature of the food before serving. Food that is too hot to eat can be cooled quickly by placing it in the freezer for a few seconds.

Thinning and thickening baby food

Most baby food should be a smooth texture. Different foods will have slightly different textures. For example, zucchini tends to be runny, and sweet potatoes are thick. Once your food cubes are thawed and ready to serve, you may decide that the consistency is not quite right and want to change it. You can mix different foods together to get the right texture or you can try one these tricks:

Thickeners: The quickest way to thicken baby food is to add vitamin-fortified dry cereal to it. This adds more vitamins to your baby's meal. Mashed banana, silken tofu, and yogurt are also great thickeners and appeal to many babies.

Thinners: The best way to thin baby food is to add breast milk or formula. Your baby is familiar with the taste of either breast milk or formula. Either of these thinners provides a good vitamin supplement to a baby's meal.

Kitchen Tools

Most of the tools you need to prepare baby food are already in your kitchen. Here is what you will need:

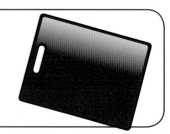

Step 1: Prep
- Cutting board
- Paring knife
- Vegetable peeler
- Spoon
- Colander or strainer

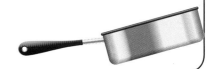

Step 2: Cook

- Potholders/oven mitts
- Saucepan and steamer basket or microwave-safe dish and cover

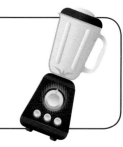

Step 3: Puree

- Blender or a food processor
- Rubber spatula or scraper

Step 4: Freeze

- Spoon or spatula
- Ice cube trays with covers or plastic wrap

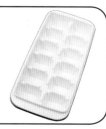

Step 5: Pop and store

- Freezer storage bags
- Permanent marker

Serving Utensils

- Bowls
- Baby spoon—the long-handled, rubber-tipped ones are ideal
- Feeding bib
- Paper towels or washcloth for cleanup

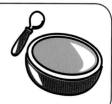

Kitchen Safety Basics

General

- All baby food should be cooked, except for bananas, tofu, and avocados.
- Clean all utensils and work surfaces before preparing baby food. Any tools that were used to handle raw foods (especially chicken, meat, or eggs) should be washed thoroughly with dish detergent and hot water.
- Wash your hands before beginning to make baby food. Make sure your hands are clean throughout the process.
- Keep hot foods hot and cold foods cold to prevent growth of bacteria. Don't let baby food sit at room temperature more than one hour. If you don't have time to put the food in freezer trays, cover it and place it in the refrigerator until later.

Preparation and Cooking

- Thoroughly wash all fruits and vegetables with water.
- Follow directions for cooking time and standing time. Stoves and microwaves vary slightly in power. Check to be sure that the food you are cooking is done. If you can easily pierce the food with a fork, it is done.
- Use only microwave-safe cookware and wraps when cooking food in the microwave.
- Wrap or cover foods completely to trap steam when cooking.

Storage

- Carefully label and date all foods that are stored in the freezer. Baby food stored in the freezer will last two months.
- Keep any leftovers in the refrigerator. Defrosted baby food will last about 2 days in the refrigerator.
- Do not save food that the baby spoon or your baby has touched.
- Discard any food that has been standing out for more than 1 hour.

Serving

- Test food for temperature before serving.
- Stir food to distribute heat evenly. If food is too hot to serve, place it in the freezer for a few seconds to cool it down.
- Use plastic or paper to serve food, even if you are spoon-feeding. It is highly likely that your baby will find some way to toss the dish or make you drop it.
- Use a spoon to feed your baby.
- Always have your baby in a sitting position for feeding. Not only is it easier to feed him, but it is also a precaution against choking. You may not be able to use a high chair for the first few months of feeding. Put your baby on your lap or in a bouncy seat or stroller.

Time Saving Tips for Making Baby Food

The homemade baby food system in this book is simple and convenient. Just set aside 30 minutes a week. You can easily make enough food to feed one baby.

Here are some tips that will help you out:

- Plan ahead. Before you go to the grocery store, look through the freezer and take inventory. Read through the recipes and select something to make. Always have a backup recipe, just in case the food you wanted to purchase is not ripe, in poor condition, unavailable, or too expensive.

- Buying frozen or canned food saves a lot of time. These foods are already washed, cleaned, and ready to cook. Washing and cleaning foods can be the most time-consuming step in the recipe.

- You can choose to cook on the stovetop or in the microwave. Pick one method and stick with it. This will help you master the technique and be more efficient.

- Plan on 30 minutes a week. Set aside the time to make your baby food. Pick a time when you do not have distractions. In the evening after your baby has gone to sleep is a great time. DON'T try to make baby food with your baby in the kitchen—it will go more slowly, it will be frustrating, and it could even be dangerous.

- Learn what your baby likes and double the recipes for her favorites. Some foods will become staples in your baby's diet. You'll save time by making twice as much.

Foods to Introduce by Age

Babies like some foods more others. With so many choices, deciding what foods to start with and when to introduce others can be tough. Here is a chart to help you decide:

First Foods (about 6 months)	6-8 Months	8-10 Months	10-12 Months	Over 12 Months
Acorn Squash	Apricots	Asparagus	Cantaloupe	Blueberries
Apples	Avocados	Lean Beef	Cherries	Raspberries
Bananas	Chicken	Black Beans	Corn	Strawberries
Butternut Squash	Nectarines	Broccoli	Eggplant	
Green Peas	Peaches	Carrots	Lamb	
Pears	Plums	Cauliflower	Pineapple	
Sweet Potatoes	Pumpkin	Garbanzo Beans (Chick Peas)		
	Turkey	Green Beans		
	Yellow Squash	Kidney Beans		
	Zucchini	Mangos		
		Papayas		
		Pinto Beans		
		Pork		
		Snow Peas		
		Spinach		
		Sugar Snap Peas		
		White Beans		
		White Potatoes		

Recipes

There are 6 basic recipes for making baby food.

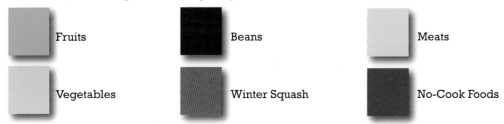

Fruits

Beans

Meats

Vegetables

Winter Squash

No-Cook Foods

The following pages provide a recipe for each kind of food.

Recipe Tips

- All quantities in the recipes are designed to make at least 24 ice-cube-sized servings of baby food (about 2 trays).

- All quantities can be easily cut in half or doubled. When doubling a recipe, cooking time may be longer.

- Fruits and vegetables vary in size. If you make too much baby food, you can:
  - Store the extra in the refrigerator; it will last for 3-4 days.
  - Store the extra in the refrigerator and freeze it in the trays the next day or when the trays have been emptied.
  - Use it for the rest of the family—they all taste great and are good for you!

- If you choose to cook food in the microwave, use only microwave-safe containers. The best choices are ceramic and lead-free glass containers or plastic that is specifically labeled "Microwave Safe"

- Cooking times might not be exact. Each recipe has a test for doneness. If the food is not quite done, try cooking 3 to 5 minutes longer and check again.

- At least once during the puree process, stop the appliance and scrape down the sides of the bowl with a spatula.

- When pureeing, add water to develop a smooth texture. The best way to add water is through the pour hole of the blender or food processor while it is pureeing. If your appliance does not have a pour hole, STOP the appliance, remove the lid, add water, secure the lid, and continue to puree.

- Frozen baby food will last 2 to 3 months in the freezer.

FRUITS

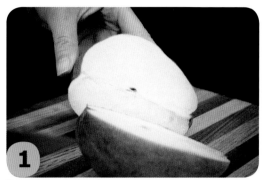

1

Prep: Wash, Peel and remove core.
Cut into pieces.

Pears

(photo example)

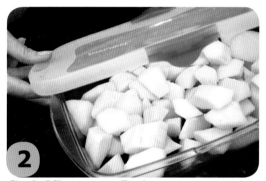

2

Cook: Microwave - 5 minutes
Stove top - 10 minutes

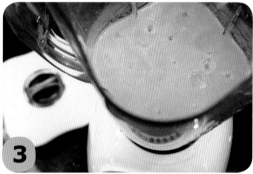

3

Puree: Blend until smooth

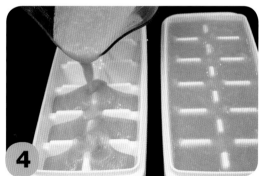

4

Freeze: Pour into trays. Cover and freeze
overnight.

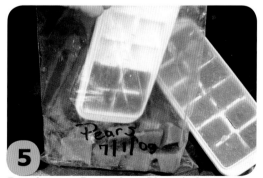

5

Pop & store: Pop cubes. Place in bag.
Return to freezer.

Fruits:

Age	Fruit	Fresh Quantity	Preparation	Cooking Time Stove / Microwave
About 6 Months	Apples	6 medium	Peel and remove core	10 min. / 5 min.
	Pears	6 medium	Peel and remove core	10 min. / 5 min.
6-8 Months	Apricots	12-14	Peel and remove pit	5 min. / 3 min.
	Nectarines	8 medium	Peel and remove pit	5 min. / 3 min.
	Peaches	6-7 large	Peel and remove pit	5 min. / 3 min.
	Plums	8-10 large	Peel and remove pit	5 min. / 3 min.
8-10 Months	Mangos	4	Peel and cut meat away from pit	5 min. / 3 min.
	Papayas	4 small or 1 X-Large	Cut in half, remove seeds with spoon, and peel	5 min. / 3 min.
10-12 Months	Cantaloupe	1 medium	Cut in half, remove seeds with spoon, and peel	5 min. / 3 min.
	Sweet Cherries	1½ pounds	Cut in half and remove pit	5 min. / 3 min.
	Pineapple	1 medium	Cut off top, bottom, and skin and remove core	5 min. / 3 min.
Over 12 Months	Blueberries	1½ pounds	Remove stems and dirt	5 min. / 3 min.
	Raspberries	1½ pounds	Remove stems and dirt	5 min. / 3 min.
	Strawberries	1½ pounds	Remove stems and dirt	5 min. / 3 min.

Quantity
Fresh Fruit: Follow the quantity information provided in the table.
Frozen Fruit: 20-25 ounces
Canned Fruit: 20-25 ounces

1. Prep
Fresh Fruits: Wash the fruit and follow the preparation instructions in the table for the fruit that you are cooking. Cut the fruit into 1-inch chunks or slices.
Frozen Fruits: Open the package and proceed to the next step.
Canned fruits: Open the cans and pour the fruit into a colander or strainer. Rinse under cold water for one minute and skip to the puree step.

2. Cook
Stove Method: Pour 1 cup of water in a large saucepan. Set a steamer basket in the saucepan. Place the fruit pieces in the steamer basket. Cover the saucepan and place on a stove burner. Set the burner temperature to HIGH and bring the water to a boil. Reduce heat to low and simmer for the suggested cooking time in the table. Let stand for 5 minutes. The fruit is done if a fork slides easily into it or it can be mashed easily. Place the fruit and 2 to 4 Tablespoons of cooking juice into a blender or food processor.

Microwave Method: Place the fruit in a microwave-safe dish. Cover with a lid. Cook on HIGH for suggested cooking time in the table. Let stand for 5 minutes. The fruit is done if a fork slides easily into it or it can be mashed easily. Place the fruit and the cooking juice into a blender or food processor.

3. Puree
Puree in the blender or food processor to a smooth texture. At least once during the puree process, stop the appliance and scrape down the sides of the bowl with a spatula.

4. Freeze
Pour or spoon the pureed fruit into ice cube trays and cover them. Put them in the freezer for 8 to 10 hours or overnight.

5. Pop and Store:
Write the type of fruit and the date on a freezer storage bag. Remove the baby food trays from the freezer and quickly run hot water over the back of the tray. Twist the tray to pop the fruit cubes out and into the freezer storage bag. Place the storage bag in the freezer.

Makes: About 24 one-ounce servings

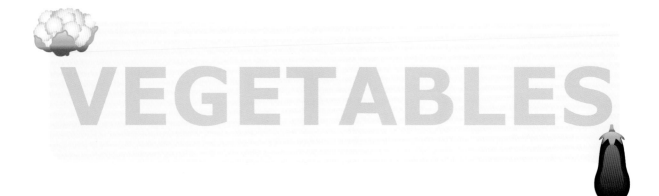

VEGETABLES

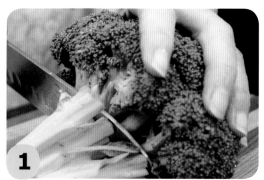

1

Prep: Wash. Cut off bottoms and chop into pieces.

Broccoli

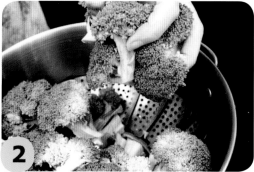

2

Cook: Stove - 10-12 minutes or microwave - 8-10 minutes.

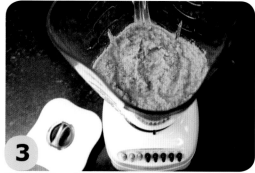

3

Puree: Blend with ¼ cup water until smooth. Add water as needed.

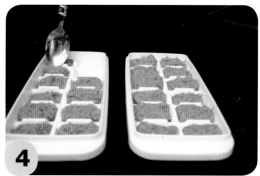

4

Freeze: Spoon into trays. Cover and freeze overnight.

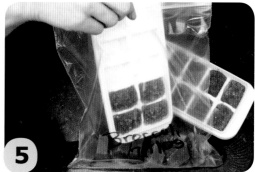

5

Pop & Store: Pop cubes. Place in bag. Return to freezer.

Vegetables:

Age	Fruit	Fresh Quantity	Preparation	Cooking Time Stove / Microwave
About 6 Months	Green Peas	1½ pounds	Shell peas and discard pods	8-10 min. /6-8 min.
	Sweet Potatoes	2-3 large	Peel	12-15 min. / 8-10 min.
6-8 Months	Yellow Squash	6-8 medium	Peel	10-12 min. /8-10 min.
	Zucchini	6-8 medium	Peel	10-12 min. /8-10 min.
8-10 Months	Asparagus	1½ pounds	Snap off tough ends and peel stalks	8-10 min. / 6-8 min.
	Broccoli	1½ pounds	Cut off bottoms	10-12 min. /8-10 min.
	Carrots	1½ pounds	Cut off both ends and peel	5 min. / 3 min.
	Cauliflower	1 medium head	Remove all leaves and core	10-12 min. / 8-10 min.
	Green Beans	1½ pounds	Remove both ends	10-12 min. / 8-10 min.
	Snow Peas	1½ pounds	Remove both ends	8-10 min. / 6-8 min.
	Sugar Snap Peas	1½ pounds	Remove both ends	8-10 min. / 6-8 min.
	Spinach	2 pounds	Remove tough stems	8-10 min. / 6-8 min.
10-12 Months	Corn	8 ears	Remove husk, wash, cut kernels off cob, discard cob	8-10 min. / 6-8 min.
	Eggplant	2-3 medium or 1 large	Peel	10-12 min. / 8-10 min.

Quantity
Fresh Vegetables: Follow the quantity information provided in the table.
Frozen Vegetables: 20-25 ounces
Canned Vegetables: 20-25 ounces

1. Prep
Fresh Vegetables: Wash the vegetables and follow the preparation instructions in the table for the vegetable that you are cooking. Cut the vegetables into 1-inch chunks or slices.
Frozen Vegetables: Open the package and proceed to the next step.
Canned Vegetables: Open the cans and pour the vegetables into a colander or strainer. Rinse under cold water for one minute and skip to the puree step.

2. Cook
Stove Method: Pour 1½ cups of water in a large saucepan. Put a steamer basket in the saucepan. Place the vegetable pieces in the steamer basket. Cover the saucepan and place it on a stove burner. Set the burner temperature to HIGH and bring the water to a boil. Reduce heat to low and simmer for the suggested cooking time in the table. Don't let the water boil away. Check the water level during cooking and add more water if needed. Let stand for 5 minutes. The vegetable is done if a fork slides easily into it or it can be mashed easily. Place the vegetables and 4 Tablespoons of cooking juice into a blender or food processor.

Microwave Method: Place the vegetables in a microwave-safe dish with 2 Tablespoons of water. Cover with a lid. Cook on HIGH for the suggested cooking time in the table. Let stand for 5 minutes. The vegetables are done if a fork slides easily into them or they can be mashed easily. Place the vegetables, cooking juice, and 2 Tablespoons of water into a blender or food processor.

3. Puree
Puree in the blender or food processor to a smooth texture. You may need to add ¼ to ½ cup of additional water to get a smooth texture. At least once during the puree process, stop the appliance and scrape down the sides of the bowl with a spatula.

4. Freeze
Pour the pureed vegetables into ice cube trays and cover them. Put them in the freezer for 8 to 10 hours or overnight.

5. Pop and Store:
Write the type of vegetable and the date on a freezer storage bag. Remove the baby food trays from the freezer and quickly run hot water over the back of the tray. Twist the tray to pop the vegetable cubes out and into the freezer storage bag. Place the storage bag in the freezer.

Makes: About 24 one-ounce servings

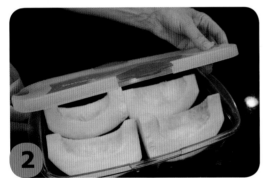

Acorn Squash

(photo example)

Prep: Wash, Cut in half, remove seeds and pierce skin with fork.

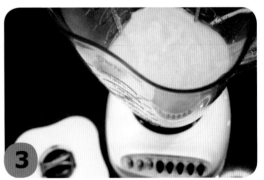

Cook: Oven - 45 minutes or Microwave - 13 -15 minutes

Puree: Blend with ½ cup water until smooth. Add water as needed.

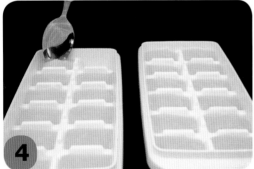

Freeze: Spoon into trays. Cover and freeze overnight.

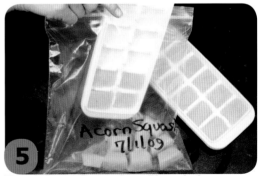

Pop & Store: Pop cubes. Place in bag. Return to freezer.

Winter Squash:

Quantity
Fresh winter squash comes in many varieties and sizes. Here are quantities for the most common types:

Acorn Squash: 1 large or 2 medium
Butternut Squash: 1 medium to large
Pumpkin*: 1 small to medium

1. Prep
Wash, cut in half, and remove seeds with a spoon. If the squash is large, cut the halves in half, making 4 pieces.

2. Cook
Oven Method: Preheat oven to 350 degrees. Place squash halves face down in a roasting pan. Pierce the squash with a fork 2 or 3 times. Pour ½ cup of water in the bottom of the pan. Bake for 45 minutes. The squash is done if a fork slides easily into it or it can be mashed easily. Let cool.

Microwave Method: Place the squash in a microwave-safe dish. Pierce the squash with a fork 2 or 3 times. Pour ½ cup of water in the bottom of the dish. Cover with a lid. Cook on HIGH for 13 -15 minutes. Let stand for 5 minutes. The squash is done if a fork slides easily into it or it can be mashed easily. Let cool.

3. Puree
Scoop squash meat away from the skin into the bowl of a blender or food processor. Discard the skin. Add ½ cup of water and begin to puree. You may need to add ¼ to ¾ cup of water to get a smooth texture. At least once during the puree process, stop the appliance and scrape down the sides of the bowl with a spatula.

4. Freeze
Pour or spoon the pureed squash into ice cube trays and cover them. Put them in the freezer for 8 to 10 hours or overnight.

5. Pop and Store:
Write the type of squash and the date on a freezer storage bag. Remove the baby food trays from the freezer and quickly run hot water over the back of the tray. Twist the tray to pop the squash cubes out and into the freezer storage bag. Place the storage bag in the freezer.

Makes: About 24 one-ounce servings

*See no-cook recipes for canned pumpkin

White Beans

(photo example)

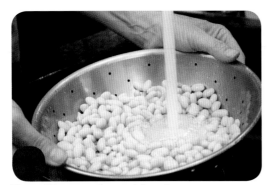

Prep: Rinse under cold water one minute.

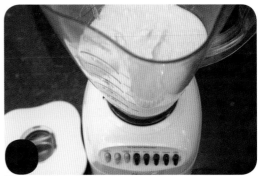

Puree: Blend with ½ cup water until smooth. Add water as needed.

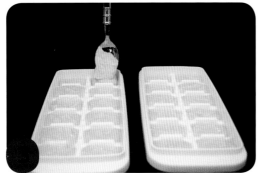

Freeze: Spoon into trays. Cover and freeze overnight.

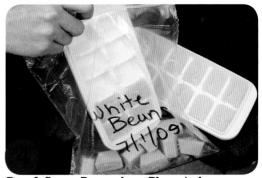

Pop & Store: Pop cubes. Place in bag. Return to freezer.

Beans:

Quantity
28 ounces (2 14-ounce cans) of any type of beans

1. Prep
Open the cans and pour the beans into a colander or strainer. Rinse under cold water for one minute.

2. Puree
Place the beans and ½ cup of water into a blender or food processor. Puree the food adding ¼ to ½ cup of water to get a smooth texture. At least once during the puree process, stop the appliance and scrape down the sides of the bowl with a spatula.

3. Freeze
Spoon the pureed beans into ice cube trays and cover them. Put them in the freezer for 8 to 10 hours or overnight.

4. Pop and Store:
Write the type of bean and the date on a freezer storage bag. Remove the baby food trays from the freezer and quickly run hot water over the back of the tray. Twist the tray to pop the bean cubes out and into the freezer storage bag. Place the storage bag in the freezer.

Makes: About 24 one-ounce servings

No-Cook Foods:

Bananas:

Prep: Slice off a piece of ripe banana and peel.

Puree: Mash with a fork. Add a little water to get a smooth texture.

Storage: Best served fresh. Save remaining banana (with the skin on) by covering the cut end with plastic wrap and storing in the refrigerator. Before using again, slice off the cut end, which may be a little brown.

Avocados:

Prep: Slice a ripe avocado in half, remove the pit, and peel off the skin.

Puree: Mash with a fork. Add a little water to get a smooth texture.

Storage: Best served fresh. Avocado cannot be frozen. You can save half the avocado for one day by leaving the pit in and keeping the peel on. Cover the avocado with plastic wrap and store it in the refrigerator.

Pumpkin:

Quantity
24 ounces 100% canned Pumpkin. Read the ingredient label and choose only 100% pumpkin puree.

Freeze
Spoon the pumpkin puree from the can into ice cube trays and cover them. Put them in the freezer for 8 to 10 hours or overnight.

Pop and Store
Write "pumpkin" and the date on a freezer storage bag. Remove the baby food trays from the freezer and quickly run hot water over the back of the tray. Twist the tray to pop the pumpkin cubes out and into the freezer storage bag. Place the storage bag in the freezer.

MEATS

Chicken

(photo example)

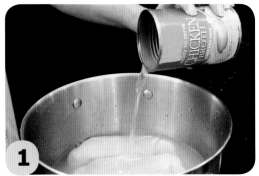

1 Cook: Stove - 15 - 20 minutes with chicken broth. Cool and chop into small pieces.

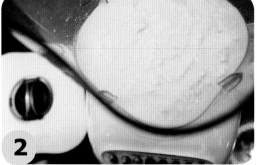

2 Puree: Blend with ½ cup broth until smooth. Add broth as needed.

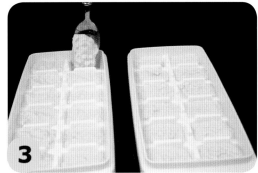

3 Freeze: Spoon into trays. Cover and freeze overnight.

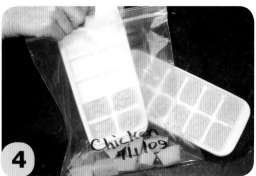

4 Pop & Store: Pop cubes. Place in bag. Return to freezer.

Chicken:

- 3 Boneless chicken breasts or 6-8 boneless chicken thighs
- 1 can (14oz.) low-sodium chicken broth

1. Cook
Place chicken in a pot with low-sodium chicken broth. Bring the pot to a boil over high heat. Turn down to low heat, cover and simmer until the chicken is done, about 15 to 20 minutes. Do not let the water boil off; add more water if necessary. To test whether it is done, remove a piece of chicken and cut it in half. If it is thoroughly cooked, the chicken meat will be white or light brown all the way through. Let chicken cool and chop into small pieces.

2. Puree
Put the chicken pieces and ½ cup of the cooking juice or chicken stock in a blender or food processor. Puree the food, adding an additional ¼ to ½ cup of cooking juice or chicken stock to get a smooth texture. At least once during the puree process, stop the appliance and scrape down the sides of the bowl with a spatula.

3. Freeze
Spoon the pureed chicken into ice cube trays and cover them. Put them in the freezer for 8 to 10 hours or overnight.

3. Pop and Store:
Write "chicken" and the date on a freezer storage bag. Remove the baby food trays from the freezer and quickly run hot water over the back of the tray. Twist the tray to pop the chicken cubes out and into the freezer storage bag. Place the storage bag in the freezer.

Makes: About 24 one-ounce servings

Beef

(photo example)

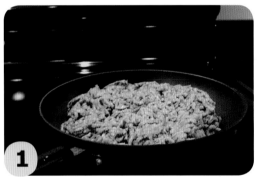

Cook: Stove - 7 - 10 minutes. Drain fat.

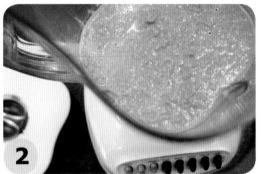

Puree: Blend with ½ cup broth until smooth. Add broth as needed.

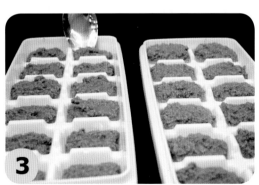

Freeze: Spoon into trays. Cover and freeze overnight.

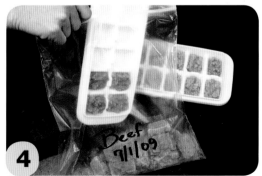

Pop & Store: Pop cubes. Place in bag. Return to freezer.

Turkey, Pork, Beef or Lamb:

- 1½ pounds of ground turkey, beef, pork, or lamb
- ½ - ¾ cup of low-sodium soup broth
    o Chicken broth for turkey and pork
    o Beef broth for beef and lamb

1. Cook
Over medium heat, add meat to a medium size non-stick skillet. Cook the meat, breaking up pieces with a wooden spoon or spatula, until completely done. Drain off any fat.

2. Puree
Place the meat and ½ cup of broth in a blender or food processor. Puree the food adding an additional ¼ to ½ cup of broth to get a smooth texture. At least once during the puree process, stop the appliance and scrape down the sides of the bowl with a spatula.

3. Freeze
Spoon the pureed meat into ice cube trays and cover them. Put them in the freezer for 8 to 10 hours or overnight.

4. Pop and Store:
Write the type of meat and the date on a freezer storage bag. Remove the baby food trays from the freezer and quickly run hot water over the back of the tray. Twist the tray to pop the meat cubes out and into the freezer storage bag. Place the storage bag in the freezer.

Makes: About 24 one-ounce servings

Stage 2 and 3 Foods:

Once your baby has been introduced to a variety of foods using the "one at a time" method, she will be ready for the next step. You can begin making meals more interesting by mixing different food cubes. You can create many different tasty combinations. Here are some ideas to get you started:

Vegetables

- Peas & sweet potatoes

- Green beans & carrots

- Carrots & peas

- Asparagus & cauliflower

- Broccoli, cauliflower, & carrots

- Butternut squash & corn

- Yellow squash & cauliflower

- Zucchini & corn

Fruits

- Peaches & pears

- Raspberries & apples

- Nectarines & bananas

- Papayas & pineapple

- Blueberries & pears

- Strawberries, peaches, & bananas

- Cantaloupe & mangos

Fruit & Vegetable Combos

- Sweet potatoes & apples

- Acorn squash & pears

- Pineapple & green beans

- Avocados & butternut squash

- Pears & peas

Vegetables & Beans

- White beans & peas

- Pinto beans & spinach

- Chick peas & broccoli

- Kidney beans & carrots

- Black beans, zucchini, & corn

Vegetables & Meat

- Chicken, broccoli, & cauliflower

- Chicken & sweet potatoes

- Chicken, corn, & peas

- Turkey & peas

- Turkey, pears, & cherries

- Beef, peas, & sweet potatoes

- Beef, corn, & green beans

- Beef & asparagus

- Pork, carrots, & cauliflower

- Pork & apples

Finger foods and textures

When your baby is between 8 and 9 months, you can introduce finger foods to encourage him to begin self-feeding. Finger foods are just as simple to make as other baby food. Choose any of the fruits or vegetables mentioned in this book. Simply cut them into cubes or spears, cook them in the microwave or steam them on the stove, and freeze them in your ice cube trays

Here are some examples of cooked finger foods:
- Apples or pear slices
- Asparagus spears
- Carrot circles or sticks
- Zucchini or yellow squash circles
- Broccoli florets
- Whole green beans

Some finger foods can be served raw, including:
- Bananas
- Avocados
- Semi-hard cheeses, such as Mozzarella, Cheddar, Jack, and Colby

At about the same time as you begin introducing finger foods (8 to 9 months), you can also begin introducing different textures in your baby's food. Lumpier and chewier foods help form your baby's (oral) mouth skills and build muscle tone. You can start with tiny, soft, almost unnoticeable lumps in your baby's foods. At first, he may spit out these lumps. In time, though, he will be able to swallow these little lumps. Slowly, you can move to introducing mashed, ground, or chopped table foods.   Examples of foods that can be mixed with baby food to add texture are:
- Fork-mashed banana, avocado, or tofu
- Puffed rice cereal
- Iron-fortified baby cereal
- Oatmeal
- Cooked rice
- Baked potato (no skin)
- Cooked pastina (or very small, mashed pieces of pasta)
- Melted cheese
- Cream of Wheat
- Grits

Feeding Memories and Fun

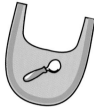

First Meal

My First Baby Food:————————————————

Age:————————

My Favorites:————————————————

Breakfast: ————————————————
————————————————

Lunch: ————————————————
————————————————

Dinner:————————————————

First Holiday:

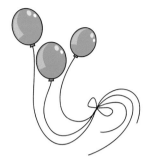

My first holiday: _____

Age: _____

Menu: _____

_____

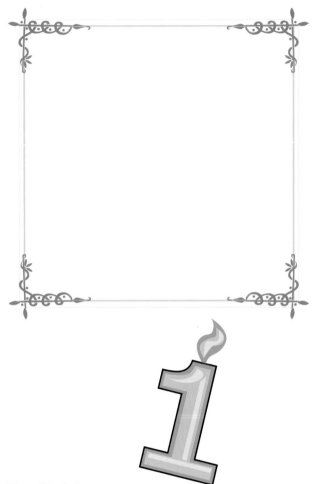

First Birthday:

Menu: _____

_____

_____